# AYURVEDA

*A Complete Ayurvedic Guide To Self-Healing And Improved Health*

## DR. JOSEPH SHIVAN

# AYURVEDA

*A Complete Ayurvedic Guide To Self-Healing And Improved Health*

## Dr. Joseph Shivan

# INTRODUCTION

**What is Ayurveda?**

Ayurveda is a holistic system of medicine that originated in India thousands of years ago. It uses a constitutional model, which aims at providing guidance regarding lifestyle and diet so that healthy individuals can stay healthy and those with illnesses can get rid of their health problem.

## Origin

Ayurveda is an intricate system of healing. It is more than just a medical system. It is considered the Science of Life. Human beings are a part and parcel of nature. Just like the plants and animals that live in harmony with the nature and follow the inherent laws of Nature to create balance within their beings, we humans, too, adhere to the principles of Mother Nature. Therefore, to say that Ayurveda helps sustain and improve the health of a person by using the basic principles of nature is justified. This system helps bring the sick individuals back to equilibrium with their true self.

In essence, Ayurveda is in existence ever since the beginning of time as all living beings including humans have always been guided and controlled by the nature's laws. Historical evidence of Ayurveda can be found in the ancient books of wisdom called the Vedas. In the Rig Veda, more than 60 preparations of natural herbs were mentioned, which could be used in overcoming various diseases. Though the Rig Veda is estimated to be written more than 6,000 years ago, Ayurveda has been around since much earlier than that.

## Meaning of Ayurveda

The word 'Ayurveda' is made up of two Sanskrit words; 'Ayu' meaning 'life' and 'Veda' meaning 'the knowledge of'. So, Ayurveda means "To know the life'. However, to fully comprehend the wide scope of Ayurveda, let us first understand life or 'Ayu'. According to Charaka, the ancient Ayurvedic scholar, "Ayu" is a combination of four vital parts – mind, body, soul and the senses.

## Mind, Body and Senses

We tend to identify only with our physical bodies; though, in reality, there is much more to us than what meets the eyes. We often ignore the mind, which underlies our physical structure. The mind not only controls our thought processes; but also assists us in carrying out our daily activities including digestion, respiration, circulation and elimination. The body and the mind work in conjunction with each other to regulate our system. In order for the mind to work appropriately for assisting the body, we use our senses for information gathering. You can think of the mind as a computer, which receives its data from the senses. For example; taste and smell are the senses that assist us in the digestive process. When the mind registers that food is entering the stomach, it passes the information to the body to act accordingly for releasing various digestive juices. Maintaining the clarity of senses is an integral part for allowing the body and mind to integrate their functions and to help us stay healthy.

## Soul

Ayurveda believes that before we exist in a physical form combined with the mind and senses; we exist in a more subtle form that is called soul. Ayurveda hypothesizes that we are comprised of an energetic essence, which precludes the inhabitance of our physical entity. We may occupy many physical bodies throughout the course of time; but our soul or the underlying self remains unchanged. Let's illustrate this concept by understanding what transpires at the time of death. When an individual nears the time to leave the physical body, most of his or her desires cease to exist. At this time, the soul no longer identifies with the body and the desire to indulge in a particular activity that used to be a source of satisfaction drops by the wayside. In fact, many individuals have documented to have experienced the sensation of being "out of their bodies."

## There are many aspects to Ayurveda which are quite unique:

- The recommendations of Ayurveda regarding which foods and lifestyle he or she should follow in order to stay healthy are often different for each patient. This is due to the constitutional model of treatment it follows.

- Everything in Ayurveda is validated by inquiry, direct examination, observation and knowledge about herbs and spices derived from the ancient texts.

- It believes that there are some energetic forces around us that influence the nature and health of human beings. These energetic forces are referred to as the Tridoshas.

- Ayurveda sees a strong connection between the mind, soul and the body. Hence, it provides a huge amount of information regarding this relationship and its effect on the mental, intellectual and physical health of a person.

## Objective of Ayurveda

This discipline has two complementary aims. The first is to maintain the health and wellbeing of individuals who are well by recommending specific diet and nutrition, lifestyle habits, hygiene, exercises and stabilizing techniques. These guidelines enable a person to maintain health and increase his or her life-span. The second one is to cure the ailments of those who are sick. This aspect relates to various disorders, their causes, diagnosis and the therapies to cure them and to prevent a relapse in future.

Both of these aims are interconnected and comprehensive areas in their own right. The primary focus of this system is to maintain your health from the outset. This is done on a daily basis to help the mind and body to be clean and stable. In this way, infections and other diseases do not find ground for establishment and aggravation.

Ayurveda aims to achieve complete health for a patient and not just to suppress his or her physical symptoms. The approach is to detect the main cause of the illness and remove it from the roots thereby allowing complete healing to occur.

The understanding of ayurveda that we are all unique individuals enables this system to address the specific health concerns of patients while offering explanation to why one patient responds differently than another. We hope you will continue exploring Ayurveda to enhance the balance of your mind, body, senses and soul and gain further insights into the beautiful miracle that we call life.

# Chapter One

# BASIC PRINCIPLES OF AYURVEDIC MEDICINE

Now that we have a more clear understanding of what our life is comprised of, let's have a look at the basic principles of Ayurveda and how they affect us.

## What is the Philosophy and Principles of Ayurvedic Medicine?

According to Ayurveda, each person is viewed as a unique individual who is made up of 5 primary elements including air, space, water, fire and earth. We derive these elements from the nature. The weather and the food we eat are the examples of the presence of these elements in the nature. When any of these elements are in an imbalance in the environment, they, in turn, have an adverse influence on us. Besides these five basic elements, there are certain other elements that seem to have an ability to create and support various physiological functions in our body.

. . .

## The 3 Doshas in Ayurveda

The 5 basic elements combine to form the three doshas or bio-energies - vata, pitta and kapha – that form the base for the treatment in Ayurveda. Ayurveda believes that the functioning of all the nature's creations including human beings, plants and animals can be understood as the interactions of these 3 basic doshas or energy complexes. The three energies together signify the mobile or dynamic, non-material, transformative, energetic, intelligent, structural and physical aspects of nature.

Firstly, air and space combine to form what is called the Vata dosha in Ayurveda. The word Vata stems from the Sanskrit word 'Vayu', which means 'something that moves'. It is considered the most influential dosha because it is the moving force behind kapha and pitta. It controls the principle of movement and is seen as a force, which directs the functions including circulation, nerve impulses, respiration and elimination. Vata energy is said to be predominant in people who are creative, lively and have a flare for innovation. A vata-dominant person is alert, quick and restless. She or he may talk, walk and think quickly; but, may also show the signs of nervousness, fear and anxiety. When out-of-balance, this energy can cause joint pains, dry skin, constipation and anxiety.

The other 2 elements - Fire and water - combine to form the Pitta dosha, which guides the process of metabolism or transformation. The term Pitta originates from the Sanskrit word 'Pinj', which means 'to shine'. This dosha is believed to add luster to the eyes, hair and the skin. The conversion of food into nutrients so that the body can use it as an energy source is an example of a pitta function. Pitta is also responsible for the metabolism in the tissue systems and organs. Pitta is also thought to control the endocrinal functions. People with pitta energy are intelligent, aggressive achievers, fiery in temperament and fast-paced. Pitta-dominant people also enjoy a hearty appetite and an efficient metabolism. But, when this energy is out of balance, it can lead to inflammation, ulcers, anger, heartburn, digestive problems and arthritis.

Finally, it is the earth and water elements that combine to form the Kapha dosha. Kapha is a term derived from the Sanskrit word 'Shlish', which means 'something that holds things together'. It governs immunity and the processes of self-repair and healing. This dosha is responsible for the growth of structures unit by unit. Kapha also offers protection to the body tissues. Cerebrospinal fluid that protects the brain and the spinal column and the mucosal lining of the stomach that protects the gastric tissues are the forms of Kapha in the body. It offers physical endurance and psychological strength while promoting human emotions like love, forgiveness, compassion, understanding, empathy, loyalty and patience. Kapha-dominant people are tenacious but calm, strong but loving and are blessed with wise tolerance. But, when this energy is out of balance, it can result in obesity, diabetes, insecurity, sinus problems and gallbladder diseases.

Our body and mind are in balance when all these three doshas are in the right proportions. Optimal health is achieved when these doshas are in harmony with the soul, senses and intellect.

. . .

The body of each person is comprised of a unique proportion of Vata, Pitta and Kapha. This is the reason for why Ayurveda sees each patient as a different individual with a special mixture, which accounts for our diversity. Hence, it designs a unique treatment protocol to specifically address a person's health challenges. When any of these doshas becomes excessive, Ayurveda suggests specific nutritional guidelines and lifestyle to help the patient in decreasing the dosha that has accumulated. Ayurveda may also advise certain herbal medications to hasten the balancing process.

An imbalance can also occur when one or more of these elements are altered qualitatively. All kinds of situations that humans experience including a thought, the climate, an emotion, food or lifestyle can have an impact on the physiological functions of the body.

**What is 'Panchakarma'?**

'Panchakarma' is the therapy of Purification. Panchakarma is recommended when there is an accumulation of harmful toxins in the body. It is a cleansing process that helps to eliminate these unwanted toxins. It is a five-fold purification therapy, which forms the classical method of treatment in ayurveda. These specialized procedures comprise of the following:

- Vaman (Therapeutic vomiting)
- Virechan (Purgation)
- Basti (Enema)
- Nasya (Elimination of toxins through the nose)

- Rakta moksha (Bloodletting or detoxification of the blood)

**What is Prakruti?**

We already learnt that, in a human body, the three doshas interact in a compensatory and harmonious way to control and sustain life. Their relative expression in a person implies a unique proportion of these bio-energies based on his or her unique DNA structure determined at conception. This is called Prakruti or the body typing of a person.

Prakruti is the specific constitution that people are born with. It can be viewed as a unique combination of psychological and physical characteristics that determine the way the person functions. Throughout life, the underlying Prakruti of an individual remains the same. However, it is constantly influenced by various internal and external factors like seasonal changes, day and night, lifestyle choices and diet. Ayurveda places emphasis on the prevention of illnesses, by maintaining health through seasonal and lifestyle regimens, which help create balance.

The implication of Prakruti helps explain why patients react in a different way to the same things. The medical application of this is certain people have a natural sensitivity to certain medicines, which results in them developing certain side effects, while others react to the same medicines in a positive way leading to complete cure of the illness.

*Chapter Two*

# DIAGNOSTIC METHODS IN AYURVEDA

Diagnosis is a very vital aspect of every system of medicine. Ayurveda, too, places a lot of emphasis on diagnosing the illness and the root cause of the same. Ayurveda, besides relieving the physical symptoms of the disease, also treats the person as a whole. Unless a proper diagnosis of the condition is done, it is difficult to begin an appropriate treatment and to cure the disease completely.

## The concept of causative factors in Ayurveda

In Ayurveda, the diagnosis of a disease is individual to each patient. The root cause of any illness may be internal or external and often varies among different individuals. All the causative factors of the disorder, directly or indirectly, create an imbalance in the three doshas i.e. Vata, Pitta and Kapha, due to which the person starts experiencing the unpleasant symptoms. The factors affecting the health can be faulty diet, lifestyle or daily activities. To give long lasting relief, this root cause has to be removed.

. . .

### Diagnostic tools in Ayurveda

Ayurveda uses five types of tools for evaluating a condition. These 5 techniques are called Pancha Nidana; 'Pancha' meaning 'five' and 'Nidana' meaning 'diagnostic methods'. These 5 methods are nidana (the cause), purva rupa (preliminary signs), rupa (symptoms), upashaya (exploratory methods) and samprapti (disease development). Now let's take a deeper look at the 5 diagnostic methods in Ayurveda.

### Nidana – The Causative factor

Nidana is the factor that causes the disease. Several factors like diet, lifestyle, injuries or environmental variations that can disturb the doshas fall in this category. Indentifying the specific foods or particular activities that can aggravate a dosha can help us avoid those triggering factors and thereby prevent the occurrence or relapse of the disease. Ayurveda gives a lot of importance to 'Nidana parivarjana' which means 'avoiding the cause'. It is considered the first line of treatment for most of the diseases.

### Purvarupa – The preliminary indications

Purva rupa means the initial signs of a disease. These symptoms start appearing much before the actual onset of the illness and often serve as a warning sign that the disease may manifest soon. Most diseases have specific set of preliminary signs. For example, in patients with epilepsy, the signs include feeling of any abnormal taste or odor, dimness of vision and a throbbing sensation all over the body.

### Rupa – The Symptoms

Rupa indicates the actual manifestation of the illness. The

disease becomes more pronounced when the obvious and clearly defined symptoms start appearing. The rupa is considered an advanced form of the purva rupa (warning signs). The number and the severity of the symptoms provide the physician a clue for predicting the physical impact of the illness, the possibility of cure (prognosis) and the length of time needed for complete healing to take place.

## Upashaya – The Exploratory Treatment

Certain diseases have similar causes, warning signs and symptoms. For example, fever can be a sign of malaria, dengue, typhoid or pneumonia. In ancient times, when the modern diagnostic techniques were not available, the diagnosis was aided by upashaya. It involves the detection and elimination of diseases through changes in diet, physical therapies and herbal remedies, which help to confirm the diagnosis.

For example, in the case of fever, the doctor often starts the treatment with Quinine to see if the symptoms are relieved. If this is achieved, it confirms that the patient had malaria. If patient does not respond to Quinine, malaria can be ruled out. Similarly, dietary changes can also be recommended to confirm an opinion about a suspected diagnosis.

## Samprapti - Development of a disease

The word Samprapti comes from 'Samyak', which means 'proper' and 'Prapti', which means 'to get'. Samprapti means to have the proper knowledge of the sequence of disease manifestation. It provides complete knowledge of the progression of the disease, starting from the causative factor and the doshas involved. It includes all the changes in the body occurring from the time of exposure to the cause to the actual onset of the disease and its manifestations.

**Benefits of Pancha Nidana**

Pancha Nidana aids in identifying the nature of the illness, its location and an effective mode of treatment. It also helps in the prevention of the disease by providing an understanding of the causative factor (nidana). Avoiding exposure to the causative factors and taking the right precautions can help people prevent the illness in future.

Similarly, having knowledge about the preliminary symptoms of a disease (purva rupa and rupa), can help a physician recommend steps to combat the disease at an initial stage, before it flares up and causes complications.

Similarly, the disease pathway (samprapti) and exploratory treatments (upashaya) allow an in-depth understanding of specific aspects of an illness and permit a physician to refine the treatment method in order to ensure a permanent cure. Therefore, the knowledge of Pancha Nidana is highly valuable in the diagnosis of diseases especially those having similar features.

**Here are some other methods of diagnosis used in Ayurveda for detecting the cause:**

**Pulse Diagnosis**

Pulse diagnosis is a highly effective tool used by ayurvedic practitioners for diagnosing the illness. For an ayurvedic practitioner, taking the pulse is more than just counting the beats. The health and functioning of the entire mind-body system can be determined from the pulse. It also helps in determining the imbalance of the doshas, the health of the various organs and the warning signs of potential health problems that may crop up in future.

The patient should be as close as possible to his norm to get an accurate pulse. The position of the index finger indicates the Vata dosha. If the vata is strong in the person, the index finger will feel a strong push of the pulse. A strong pulse against the middle finger indicates the Pitta dosha. When the pulse feels stronger under the ring finger, it is the sign of Kapha constitution.

**Eye Diagnosis**

Vata eyes appear small with dry, scanty lashes and drooping eyelids. The cornea looks muddy and the iris is black or gray-brown. Pitta eyes are moderate in size and appear sharp and lustrous. The lashes are oily and scanty. Kapha eyes are large and beautiful with long and thick lashes.

**Tongue Diagnosis**

A whitish tongue indicates an imbalance in Kapha while a yellowish-green or red tongue indicates a Pitta imbalance. A vata imbalance is manifested by a brown or black discoloration on the tongue.

**Facial Diagnosis**

Ayurveda believes that the face is a mirror of the mind. Mental as well as physical disorders are manifested on the face in the form of discoloration, wrinkles and lines. For example, excessive horizontal wrinkling on the forehead can be a sign of deep-seated anxieties or worries. Full and fluffy lower eyelids may point towards impaired kidneys.

The nose can be used for determining the dosha of a person. People with dominant Vata have crooked nose. People with dominant Kapha have a blunt nose and those with dominant Pitta have a sharp nose.

## Nail Diagnosis

Nails that are dry and rough indicate a predominance of Vata constitution. Pink, soft and tender nails are an indication of Pitta constitution. If the nails are strong, thick and very shiny, then Kapha predominates.

## Lip Diagnosis (OSTHA)

Dry and rough lips are an indication of vata imbalance. Repeated attacks of red patches along the margins of the lips point towards a chronic pitta derangement.

# Chapter Three

# HYPERTENSION AND AYURVEDA

Hypertension or high blood pressure has become a major cause of disability and death all over the world. If neglected, it can result in number of complications like heart attacks, cerebrovascular stroke and kidney failure. In most cases, it does not cause any apparent symptoms until these complications occur. It plays the role of silent killer in the body. Hence, it is important to keep in mind that you may have hypertension and the only way you can know about it is to get your blood pressure checked at regular intervals.

**What is hypertension?**

Hypertension means elevated pressure of the blood in the arteries. It is known as Rakta Gata Vata in Ayurveda. Normal blood pressure of a healthy adult is 120 mm of Hg systolic and 80 mm of Hg diastolic. The rise in blood pressure depends on the age, sex, family history, physical activities and diet of a person.

. . .

**Here are few Ayurvedic remedies that are effective in lowering blood pressure naturally:**

## Ashwagandha

Ashwagandha is a popular Ayurvedic herb known for its adaptogenic properties. It keeps the blood pressure within normal limits and reduces inflammation and damage in the arteries caused due to the persistent high pressure. It strengthens the mind and body and improves the ability of a person to handle psychological and physical stress thereby tackling the root cause of the illness. It also increases vitality and resistance and produces a strengthening effect on the body functions.

Stress is one of the commonest causes of high blood pressure. The excessive production of stress hormones like cortisol can result in further elevation of the blood pressure. Ashwagandha increase the person's ability to cope with stress thereby creating greater inner calmness. This, in turn, reduces the level of cortisol circulating in the body and controls blood pressure.

### Triphala

Triphala has been used since centuries for rejuvenating the body. It consists of three herbs that together form a powerful combination, which works in a profound; but gentle way. The three herbs are Haritaki (Terminalia chebula), Amla (Emblica officinalis) and Bibhitaki (Terminalia bellica).

Triphala reduces hypertension and normalizes blood circulation. It also reduces cholesterol, which is another common cause of hypertension and works towards preventing atherosclerosis. The anti-inflammatory and anti-obesity effects of this formula help in preventing hypertension by tackling the other 2 causes of the illness namely inflammation and obesity.

## Jatamansi

Jatamansi protects the arteries from the damage caused by free radicals. It repairs the arterial damage caused by cholesterol plaques and thereby improves the inner diameter of the blood vessels. This allows the blood to flow freely through the arteries, which ensures lower force created by the blood on the walls of arteries. This herb also creates a calming effect on the mind and body and hence, is highly effective in reducing psychological stress.

## Arjuna

Arjuna is a powerful herb for treating high blood pressure. It reduces the level of low density lipoprotein (bad) cholesterol in the liver and increases the production of high density lipoprotein (good) cholesterol thereby reducing the risk of atherosclerosis.

It also reduces the effects of stress and anxiety on the heart by reducing the production of stress hormones and protects the blood vessels from the damage caused by them.

These herbal remedies are based on the healing principles of Ayurveda. These herbs are safe and natural and do not cause any harmful side effects.

# Chapter Four

# DIET AND LIFESTYLE RECOMMENDATIONS

For better control of the illness and for preventing the complications, patients are advised to follow some dietary and lifestyle recommendations given below:

- Avoid meat and eggs. Reduce the intake of table salt and other food items that are high in salt like pickles. Reduce protein intake. Eat lots of fruits like melons and vegetables like Garlic, lemon and parsley.
- Avoid smoking as it increases heart rate. Smoking also worsens atherosclerosis resulting in further aggravation of the problem.
- Exercise regularly. Brisk walking, jogging and swimming are good options. Exercising also helps to control obesity, which is a common precursor of hypertension. Avoid strenuous activities if your blood pressure is very high.
- Nurture love and affection. Love and an affectionate touch can drop your blood pressure significantly.

- Laughter is the best medicine; it relieves anxiety and stress. It also emits positive energy and helps you keep negative energies at bay. Laughter works as a good relaxation therapy also. It decreases the production of stress hormones. If you are frustrated, angry or sad; just laugh and you will find yourself away from the rage. It is a very effective medicine that is always with you, without spending a penny for it.

**Meditation and Breath Therapy for Hypertension:**

You can achieve complete tranquility of the mind by meditating in the Corpse Pose. To practice this, take slow deep breaths and concentrate on the incoming and outgoing breath. Focus on the temperature of the breath while inhaling and exhaling. You may notice that the inhaled air is slightly colder than the exhaled air. Do this for 10 minutes daily to get rid of stress and the resulting high blood pressure. Research has proved that people, who practice Corpse Pose, regularly have a better control on their blood pressure.

# Chapter Five

# DIABETES AND AYURVEDA

**Diabetes Mellitus**

Diabetes Mellitus is a metabolic disorder, which affects the ability of the body to make proper use of glucose. It may occur due to the lack of Insulin produced in the pancreas (type 1 Diabetes) or because of the inability of the body to utilize the insulin efficiently (Type 2 Diabetes). The risk factors for this condition include obesity, sedentary lifestyle, family history, faulty diet and smoking. It is a chronic disorder characterized by persistent high levels of blood sugar due to the improper metabolism of carbohydrates in the body. The excess of glucose in the blood also results in increased amount of glucose being passed in the urine. This causes an increase in the urine output due to which the patient also develops dehydration and increased thirst.

**Ayurvedic View**

In Ayurveda, Diabetes Mellitus is known as Madhumeha. The word is derived from Madhu, which means 'honey' and Meha, which means 'urine'. This disorder is categorized as Vataj Meha, an imbalance caused by the excess of Vata or Air. Deterioration of the cells and tissues in the body is a characteristic feature of the impairment of Vata. This is the reason why all vital organs including the liver, the heart, the brain and the kidneys are affected due to Diabetes.

Madhumeha is considered a Maha Rog (Major Disease) because, if not treated properly, it can cause serious complications like kidney failure, stroke, heart attacks and impotency. Though it is a metabolic disorder, it can not be controlled by merely reducing the sugar levels. Ayurveda recommends treatment that is aimed at rejuvenating the whole body besides reducing the sugar level. The holistic treatment also ensures that no further complications are caused.

**Natural control of Diabetes with herbs**

There are several herbs that are highly effective in reducing the level of sugar in blood. The greatest advantage of these herbal supplements is that they cause no side effects even when used for several years. Given below is a list of some of the most effective herbs for an effective control of Diabetes.

- **Bitter Gourd**

Bitter gourd is considered the best herbal remedy for diabetes. Patients are advised to drink at least one tablespoon of bitter gourd juice daily. Alternatively, they can also add 1 tablespoon of Indian gooseberry juice to 1 cup of bitter gourd juice and take this mixture daily. This will enable the pancreas to secrete more insulin.

- **Cinnamon**

Cinnamon helps regulate blood sugar levels by correcting the metabolism of carbohydrates in the body. Research has found that this spice has the potential to lower the fasting blood glucose significantly. Regular use of Cinnamon in food preparation also helps to prevent any damage to the heart and reduces the risk of heart attacks.

- **Green Tea**

Green tea contains polyphenols that possess strong antioxidant properties. The main antioxidant in green tea, Epigallocatechin Gallate (EGCG), has numerous health benefits including improved glucose control, better insulin activity and lowered risk of cardiac complications.

- **Grapes**

Many people are surprised to know that this juicy fruit can actually help in controlling diabetes. In fact; many patients think they must avoid this fruit. But, the fact is grapes contain a chemical called Resveratrol that helps in lowering blood sugar. It can also reduce mental stress and helps in preventing sudden rise in blood sugar following stressful conditions.

- **Garlic**

Garlic or Allium Sativum offers strong antioxidant properties. The studies have proved a direct link between the regular consumption of Garlic and an effective control of diabetes. It causes a reduction in blood glucose by increasing the secretion of Insulin. It also slows down the degradation of insulin. The micro-circulatory effects of this herb help in improving the flow of blood in the vital organs of the body thereby preventing the complications caused by the lack of blood supply like stroke and peripheral vascular disorders.

- **Bauhinia Forficata**

Bauhinia Forficata has been referred to as 'vegetable insulin' because of the wonderful therapeutic effect it produces in patients suffering from Type 1 Diabetes. Regular utilization of this herb as tea infusion can help patients keep the disease in control.

- **Ivy gourd**

Ivy gourd or Coccinia Indica has been found to possess insulin-mimetic properties, which means it mimics the action of insulin. It also facilitates glucose uptake by the body so that it can be used as an energy source. Significant favorable changes in blood sugar level have been observed in studies involving this herb. Some studies have also reported regeneration of the islet cells (the pancreatic cells that regulate the carbohydrate metabolism) and an increase in beta-cell activity.

- **Milk Thistle**

Milk Thistle or Silibum Marianum contains high concentrations of antioxidants and flavonoids, which have a beneficial effect on insulin resistance. It improves the receptivity of the body cells to insulin and makes it more effective. It is widely used in the treatment of Type 2 Diabetes.

**Diet and lifestyle changes for Diabetes**

The Ayurvedic treatment for this disease is based on the entire change in the lifestyle of the person. Along with herbal medications, patients are also advised to eat nutritious food and lead a healthy lifestyle. Lifestyle and dietary changes rejuvenate the cells and tissues in the body, allowing them to produce more insulin.

Here are some dietary recommendations for diabetic patients. These recommendations can also help prevent the occurrence of the illness in those who are in the high-risk category.

- Avoid sugar in any form including rice, potato, cereals and fruits like mangoes, pineapple and banana
- Include one bitter dish in at least one meal of a day
- Eat plenty of black gram, green vegetables, fish and soy
- Eat vegetables like string beans, cucumber, bitter gourd, onion and garlic and fruits like Jambul and watermelon

## Lifestyle for Diabetes patients

- Quit smoking
- Avoid sleeping during daytime
- Exercise regularly
- Control your weight
- Take adequate eye care
- Take extra care of your foot

# Chapter Six

# TREATMENT AND APPROACH OF AYURVEDA FOR CHOLESTEROL DISORDERS

**What is hypercholesterolemia?**

Hypercholesterolemia is a disorder characterized by high level of cholesterol. Cholesterol is a soft, waxy substance found among the fats in all of the body's cells, especially in the bloodstream. It is present in small quantities and forms a part of the nerve coverings, cell walls and the brain cells. Hence, it has an important function in the body. However, when this substance is present in excess quantities, it can cause blockages in the arteries resulting in serious consequences.

**Ayurvedic treatment for managing cholesterol disorders**

Ayurvedic approach for treating this condition includes eliminating the toxins and mucus from the blood vessels and to restore the digestive fire to allow it to perform optimally for burning excess fats.

. . .

## Dangers of high cholesterol

Excessive amount of cholesterol circulating in the blood can lead to a slow build up of this substance in the walls of the arteries of the heart and brain. It combines with other substances and forms thick, hard deposits called plaque that can clog those arteries. This condition is called atherosclerosis. If the plaque breaks away in piece and circulates in blood, it can travel to distant organs like the heart or the brain causing heart attacks or stroke, respectively.

## Here are some herbs that have strong medicinal properties for lowering cholesterol:

- **Alfalfa**

Alfalfa clears the arteries congested with cholesterol by producing a disintegrating effect on the plaques. Regular consumption of this herb can help people control their cholesterol levels and avoid the complications of this condition.

- **Arjuna**

Arjuna has been used since centuries in the management of cardiac problems like heart attacks. The bark of this herb, when taken in a powder form, has beneficial medicinal properties. It can dissolve the cholesterol accumulated in the coronary arteries and reduces the risk of heart attacks.

- **Coriander**

Coriander works as an excellent diuretic. It helps to control cholesterol by boosting the functions of the kidneys. It ensures that the kidneys flush out the excess cholesterol from the body via urine thereby reducing blood cholesterol level.

- **Garlic**

Garlic is highly beneficial for people with cholesterol problems. Experts recommend eating two to three cloves of garlic everyday, first thing in the morning. It can be chewed raw if the sharp taste can be tolerated or simply gulped down with a glass of water. It helps to eliminate the cholesterol from the blood by disintegrating the plaques and frees up the arteries.

- **Guggulu**

This is a popular Indian herb, which has strong medicinal properties for treating cholesterol-related heart problems. It contains guggulsterones that help reduce the levels of cholesterol. It also has the capacity to dissolve the cholesterol plaques in the arteries so that it can be excreted via urine.

## Dietary and lifestyle changes for managing high cholesterol

Ayurveda also suggests a disciplined diet and regular exercise plan to achieve healthy levels of cholesterol. Here are a few time-tested measures that can help patients bring their cholesterol levels to normal and keep it that way.

- Start your day with high fiber grains like oats and fresh fruits. Eat plenty of dried beans or legumes and seafood especially salmon, sardine and tuna. Oysters, mussels and clams are also beneficial in lowering cholesterol.

- Eat lots of fruits concentrated in antioxidant compounds like citrus fruits, apple and strawberries. Nuts like almonds and walnut and vegetables like spinach, broccoli and carrots are also rich in antioxidant compounds.

- Drink plenty of water. This causes an increased excretion of water along with the toxins and excess fats from the body.

- Do regular exercises like brisk walking - for at least 40 minutes everyday, for 5 days a week. Regular physical activities can help control obesity and improve the body's metabolic rate, which, in turn, accelerates the utilization of excess fats.

- Keep a watch on the amount of calories you consume. Say no to red meats, chocolates, ice creams and all other foods that can increase your calorie count. Foods rich in fats like fried foods, too, should be avoided.

- Practice deep breathing exercise and meditation for 15-20 minutes daily. It helps refresh your mind and body and is also an effective de-stress technique.

- Quit smoking. Smoking increases the tendency for the blood to clot and worsens atherosclerosis. It also causes damage to the walls of the arteries. Besides this, the recovery of patients, who have suffered a heart attack due to high cholesterol, is much slower in smokers than in nonsmokers.

- Avoid excess of alcohol. People, who consume moderate amounts of alcohol, have a lower risk of cardiac complications than non-drinkers. However, increased consumption of alcohol can bring about other health dangers like high blood pressure, stroke and obesity.

# Chapter Seven

# SKIN CARE IN AYURVEDA

Skin is the largest sense organ of our body. It is also the part of the body that defines the beauty and attractiveness of a man and a woman. Skin serves as a protective barrier between our internal organs and safeguards it from any damage caused by the factors in the external environment. Skin regulates the body temperature and is in a continuous state of growth, with old cells dying and the new cells forming. The skin is affected by every aspect of our life, including what we eat, when and how much we sleep and where we live.

**Why is skin care important?**

Proper skin care is essential for all men and women who are concerned about their physical appearance. Unhealthy skin appears dull, whereas a healthy skin looks vibrant and glowing. Wrinkles develop with more ease if your skin is unhealthy and not well hydrated. An unhealthy skin also loses its elasticity faster and makes it sag and develop folds. A healthy skin has an ability to heal faster. Therefore, it is important to take proper care of your skin so that it looks radiant and exudes confidence in your personality.

### Ayurvedic approach for skin care

The holistic management of skin problems in ayurveda comprises of the three-fold approach through herbal medications, diet and lifestyle.

Ayurveda has stated that skin problems primarily occur due to the sluggish liver functions resulting in Kapha and Pitta Dosha. It causes a build up of toxins in the body and later these impurities show up as skin problems like break-outs, eczema or pigmentations. Ayurveda advises people to drink lots of water to flush out the impurities.

Another vital factor that can contribute to the healthy appearance of the skin is a clean bowel. Ayurveda stresses on the need for regular and complete evacuation of the bowels. In order to achieve this, a diet high in fibers like papaya, oranges and watermelons is recommended.

Stress is the most common cause of skin problems. The occurrence or aggravation of acne, eczema, melasma and skin cancer is largely linked to mental stress. It starts a chain of reaction resulting in dryness of the skin, loss of skin luster and wrinkle formation. Ayurveda advises people to follow the de-stressing techniques like yoga, meditation and deep breathing exercises for keeping the skin younger and healthier.

### The 3 best herbs for an attractive and vibrant skin

### 1. **Turmeric (Haldi)**

Turmeric nourishes the skin, purifies blood and gives it a natural glow. It possesses anti-aging, anti-inflammatory and anti-bacterial properties that help reduce inflammation in acne, pigmentations and blemishes and prevents infections. It also heals ulcers and wounds on the skin. It is known for its hydrating properties. It prevents dryness of the skin and keeps it soft and supple. It also slows down the skin aging process.

**How to Use:**

- On a hot day, mix 2 spoonfuls of turmeric powder in half the quantity of rice powder, tomato juice and raw milk each to make a paste. Apply it on the face and neck and leave it for 30 minutes. Rinse with lukewarm water. The skin will look brighter and fresh after this.

- You can also use it as a night cream. Prepare a paste from turmeric and yogurt or milk and apply it on your face. Leave it on overnight and wash off the mask gently in the morning with water.

- Apply a mixture of turmeric and lime juice on the exposed areas of the skin to remove tanning.

### I. **Sandalwood (Chandan)**

Sandalwood is the key ingredient in most of the Ayurvedic skin-care formulas. It is effective in treating rashes, scrapes, acne and blemishes. The paste and oil of Sandalwood, when used externally, produce a cool, calming effect on the body. It helps balance the body after overexposure to the sun and prevents sunburns. Sandalwood powder can be made into a paste for hydrating and cleansing the skin.

**How to Use:**

1. To treat acne, make a thick paste of 1 teaspoon of sandalwood powder and 1 teaspoon of turmeric. Apply the paste on the pimples before going to bed.

1. You can treat eczema by applying the mixture of sandalwood and lime juice on the affected parts. Leave it for 20-30 minutes and rinse with cool water. This will help reduce the itching and irritation of the skin.

1. Sandalwood oil is used as a moisturizer for the face. Gentle massage of the face and the body with this oil can have a rejuvenating effect on the skin. It also relaxes the muscles and makes one feel lighter; but energetic.

1. Mix four teaspoons of sandalwood powder in two teaspoons of almond oil and five tablespoons of coconut oil. Apply this mixture on the exposed parts of your skin. You will notice a significant improvement in your tan.

## 1. **Aloe Vera (Ghritkumari)**

Aloe Vera is a popular ayurvedic medication known for its anti-inflammatory and anti-fungal properties. It also possesses healing and cooling properties. It hastens the healing of acne, skin wounds, burns, scalds, insect bites, blisters and rashes. It is also used for alleviating the symptoms of allergic reactions of the skin and vaginal infection. The gel of this plant can protect the outer layer of the skin and prevent inflammation.

**How to use:**

- Apply Aloe Vera gel on the face before applying any make-up. This will help prevent the skin from drying.

- Add the pulp of some fresh fruits to Aloe Vera gel and put this in a blender to make a thick paste. Use it as a face pack to keep the skin cool.

- Mix Aloe Vera with almond oil or wheat germ and use it as a moisturizing pack.

- To treat pigmentation, cut a leaf of Aloe Vera and split it to remove the gel. Apply the gel on the skin and leave it for 10-20 minutes. Wash it off with mild soap and water.

- In case of sunburn, applying Aloe Vera gel can help create a protective barrier on the skin and replenish its moisture.

# Chapter Eight

# MEDICINAL USAGE OF HERBS & SPICES - YOUR KITCHEN PHARMACY

In a perfect world, we can get all the nutrients we need from the food we eat. But sadly we do not live in a perfect world. The food available to us has undergone a drastic change in the past century, making healthy eating a challenge. We tend to eat more of unhealthy or junk food than nutritious and healthy food though we have our spice rack filled with seasonings having excellent medicinal powers. We just grab these spices in a hurry, but do we know the healing powers these ancient herbs possess? Do we know that, when used regularly and in the right way, these kitchen spices and herbs can actually turn our kitchen into a pharmacy that has a medication for most health problems?

Much before the health stores made specific herbs readily available for therapeutic use, people relied on these culinary herbs to play a pharmaceutical role in the family.

The great thing about these spices and herbs is that most of us already have them in our kitchen, which makes the entire process less intimidating.

. . .

Using kitchen herbs is less expensive and does not require an extensive knowledge of herbal treatment. Anyone can use these herbs successfully to heal and regenerate the body. Before you begin to take a stock of your spice rack, let's learn about the common culinary herbs and spices, how to use them and their healing properties.

## Basil

Basil produces a strong antimicrobial and antioxidant activity. It stimulates the appetite and eases stomach upsets. Basil supports the kidney functions and helps in detoxifying the blood by eliminating the harmful toxins from the body via urine. Basil also sharpens memory and improves attention span and concentration power. It eases gum ulcers, earaches and itching or irritation of the skin. Use Basil leaves in soups, salads and dips. You can also saute it with greens or use it in pasta sauces.

## Ginger

Ginger has anti-inflammatory properties that protect the body against infections caused by bacteria and fungi. It also eliminates intestinal gas and soothes the intestinal tract, while boosting the immune system. It can prevent the progression of atherosclerosis by lowering cholesterol levels. Ginger also helps to overcome nausea. Ginger can be cut into smaller pieces and added to any food preparation.

## Nutmeg

Nutmeg is used to boost mental health and to reduce

anxiety. It elicits a significant antidepressant-like effect that is comparable to the antidepressants like Imipramine and Fluoxetine. It can also be used for treating insomnia, restlessness and nervousness.

## Cloves

Clove is one of the best stimulants. It is known for its vaso-relaxing properties. Cloves are rich in minerals like iron, calcium, sodium, potassium and manganese. Clove oil can be used as a local anesthetic agent for relieving toothache. It also reduces cough, asthma, bronchitis and stress.

## Cinnamon

Cinnamon contains calcium, iron and manganese. It can be used in the treatment of nutritional deficiencies like anemia. Cinnamon can be used by diabetic patients to control their blood sugar levels. It reduces digestive problems and improves brain functions.

## Parsley

Parsley's medicinal effects come from its flavonoids: apiole, terpinolene, myristicin and appin. Parsley offers therapeutic benefits in the management of renal problems like urinary tract infections and kidney stones. It is also effective in relieving gastrointestinal distress. Moreover, it can also be used to regularize menses. Use it in salads or soups as a garnish. Take care not to overcook it as the herb may lose its potency and color.

## Bay Leaf

Bay leaf acts as a stimulant for the skin. It improves the glow on the skin and makes it more firm and soft thereby preventing wrinkles. Regular use of this herb in food can help prevent rashes in patients having a sensitive skin. Use it as a flavoring agent for stews, soups, pilafs and with seafood.

## Tarragon

Tarragon works well as a de-worming agent. Parents can give this herb to their children to stave off intestinal parasites. Tarragon has also been used to treat toothaches and gastric upsets. Just like parsley, Tarragon can also be used to manage menstrual disorders like amenorrhea and dysmenorrhea. It is used in classic French sauces, vinegars and vinaigrettes. It can also be used to roast chicken.

## Dill

Dill is used to treat gastrointestinal disorders like stomach upset, flatulence, gastric ulcers and indigestion. It is also used to treat insomnia, stress and anxiety disorders. Some parents give an infusion or tea of Dill to their young babies for relieving colic. Dill is used in the preparation of pickles, fish stews and beet soups.

## Lavender

Lavender is an excellent ayurvedic medication for treating loss of appetite and insomnia. It is found to be useful in the treatment of circulatory disorders. It is often used to treat migraine, restlessness and cramps. Lavender can be used in teas, scones, cookies and sweets. It can be combined with honey, mint, oats or rose syrup for adding flavor.

## Oregano

Oregano helps in the treatment of respiratory diseases like stuffy nose and chronic cough. It works as an expectorant. It liquefies the secretions and aids in the easy expulsion of the mucus thereby relieving breathing difficulties caused due to the blockages. It is effective in relieving menstrual cramping and has potent antimicrobial activities. Oregano can be used to flavor olive oil and to season lamb and goat milk cheeses. It is also used in tomato sauces and in chilies.

### Sage

Sage is known for its healing properties for relieving inflammation, particularly of the mouth. It improves appetite and eases digestion. Nursing mothers, who experience overproduction of the milk resulting in breast engorgement, can use Sage to slow the milk production. This herb is used as a rub for pork and to roast poultry.

### Rosemary

Rosemary is used to ease headaches and migraines. It also helps to relieve stomach upsets and menstrual disorders. It can be applied externally to speed the healing of wounds and eczema. Rosemary can also help lower blood pressure in patients with hypertension. Rosemary is used in herbal vinegars and roasts.

### Peppermint

Peppermint is mostly taken as a tea or in infusions to treat colic and digestive upset. It is commonly used in the treatment of common cold and flu, thanks to its ability to open the sinuses. When used in combination with honey, it can help ease a sore throat. Peppermint essential oil can be applied on the temples to help with headaches and migraines. It is used in sweets and confections. It can also be used in the preparation of whipped cream or fruit salad and as a garnishment to roast lamb.

## Licorice

Licorice boosts the immune system and buffers the inflammatory response by stimulating the production of steroids by the adrenal glands. It also modifies the response of the immune system to fight and relieve the symptoms of infection.

# Chapter Nine

# THE AYURVEDIC FIRST AID KIT INFECTION

Children as well as adults are susceptible to incidents that can harm us and even result in minor or major injuries. So, we all keep a first aid kit ready at home packed with bandages, antiseptic cream, plasters, wipes, pain killing drugs and antacids. But, what if you want to achieve a quick first aid relief naturally? With just a little patience and proper know how, you can easily find a natural remedy from your own kitchen for administering first aid in case of emergencies. Here are few first aid natural remedies that you can use in such case:

### Sore throat

A classic combination of turmeric and honey works fast and effectively for relieving a sore throat. Just mix a spoonful of both these natural remedies and suck on the spoon. Alternatively, you can add turmeric and rock salt in warm water and do gargling. You will find an instant relief from the problem.

.  .  .

## Cuts

Applying a paste of turmeric and honey on the cut will stop the bleeding within few seconds. Just make the paste and press it on the wound. It also acts as an anti-septic and prevents any infection. It will also help the wound to heal faster. This natural tip is beneficial even for diabetic patients in whom any injury can take a longer time to heal and may result in an infection.

## Burn

The first thing to do in case of burns is to immediately run the part through cold water. Let the water flow over the part as long as the burning sensation remains. This will not only relieve the pain; but also prevent the blisters from form-ing. Then, apply a paste of Aloe Vera gel with a pinch of turmeric powder. You can leave it till the initial sting subsides. You can continue applying aloe or apply coconut oil with sandalwood or rose to enhance the cooling effect.

## Headache

Apply a paste of ginger on the forehead and lie down for about 5-10 minutes. Then, remove the paste. You will find the headache disappearing miraculously after this. The aroma of Ginger will also make you feel more refreshed. Headaches can also be a sign of dehydration. So, drink 1-2 glasses of water especially if you start getting headache after a workout or due to travelling under harsh sun. A gentle massage to the forehead, temples, shoulders and neck with Eucalyptus oil can also help loosen up the muscles and relieve the headache. Sinus headache can be relieved by applying gingelly oil mixed with camphor on the forehead.

. . .

## Acid reflux

Acid reflux is usually a result of an increase in the pitta dosha. A pitta pacifying diet can help correct this problem quickly. You can try chewing on fennel seeds or drink Aloe Vera juice to relieve the pain. You can also drink a glass of buttermilk with a pinch of fenugreek and asafetida. This will help neutralize the acid in the stomach and prevent regurgitation and the resulting heartburn.

## Indigestion

The best natural quick fix for this very common problem is drinking a glass of pomegranate juice. You can also try drinking hot water infused with lemon juice. Drinking buttermilk with cumin seeds and a little salt can help relieve flatulence and abdominal discomfort instantly.

## Cold and Cough

Dry cough can be treated by taking a decoction of liquorice root. If you suffer from cough with lot of mucous secretion, take a decoction of ginger, turmeric, pinch of black pepper, lemon and a squeeze of honey once it cools down. You can also eat a paste of garlic or chew on ginger root. You will find great relief by boiling some ginger powder in water and inhaling the steam. Applying few drops of Eucalyptus oil on the sides of the nose will help to relieve nose block. Inhaling the powder of calamus root into each nostril can also reduce the congestion.

## Diarrhea

If diarrhea is a result of indigestion or overeating, drink a glass of buttermilk with a pinch of salt and asafetida. Another great remedy for treating loose motions is powdered mango seed taken with honey. A mix of rock salt, dry ginger and jaggery is also effective in cases of diarrhea caused by indigestion.

## Acne

Acne can be an emergency sometimes. A small pimple here or there on your face can send you in a tizzy especially when it crops up before a special event. Though the pimple will not disappear completely within just a day, it can reduce in intensity and appear less visible by applying a paste of sandalwood powder and turmeric on it. Take about one teaspoon of each of these powders and mix them with rose water to make a paste. For internal treatment, drink 1 cup of fresh Aloe vera juice, two times a day, till the acne clears.

## Asthma

Combine ginger herb with Licorice and drink it as a tea. The recommended proportion is about one teaspoon of both the herbs for one cup of water. Drinking onion juice mixed with 1-2 teaspoons of honey and a pinch of black pepper can also provide relief from asthma attack.

## Backache

Gentle massage of the back with a paste of ginger and eucalyptus oil can help relieve the spasm of the muscles in the back and reduce back pain. Backache resulting from bone-related disorders can be relieved by massaging with coconut oil. However, it can only reduce the pain for a short duration and not cure the disease completely.

· · ·

## Bad breath

Drinking half a cup of Aloe Vera and eating a teaspoonful of fennel seeds can help reduce the bad breath. You can also chew on peppermint or ginger to avoid this problem.

## Bleeding

External bleeding can be arrested by applying ice or sandalwood paste. For stopping internal bleeding, patients are advised to drink warm milk with half teaspoon each of saffron and turmeric powder. This should be followed by consultation with a medical professional to ascertain the cause of bleeding so that appropriate measures can be taken.

## Toothache

Toothache can be instantly relieved by applying 2-3 drops of clove oil on the affected tooth. You can also put the drops on a piece of sterilized cotton ball and press it between the teeth. Gargling with salt water or slightly warm sesame oil can also provide relief from toothache.

## Boils

Applying a paste of ginger and turmeric powder directly on the boil or using cooked onions as a poultice can help a boil heal quickly.

## Burning in the Eyes

Put in four drops of rose water or fresh Aloe Vera juice into the affected eye. You can also apply Castor oil to the soles of the feet.

# Chapter Ten

# FOOD ANTIDOTES IN AYURVEDA

**What is antidote?**

An antidote is a substance that counteracts a particular medicine or an unpleasant sensation. Sometimes, the food we eat can cause many problems like nausea, vomiting, diarrhea, gastric trouble, skin rashes and asthma. These negative effects can occur due to overindulgence or hypersensitivity of the person to that substance.

While it is ideal to avoid overindulging too often, it is hard to give away the temptation and 'let our hair down' every now and then. Besides food items, there are several other factors like excessive exposure to the sun and travelling that can affect our will being and hence, need to be tackled appropriately. You can counter the negative effects of these things by using the natural herbs in ayurveda. Below I've listed some powerful, natural antidotes that you can use to offset the 'not so healthy' effects of certain things.

. . .

## Overindulgences & Their antidotes:
### Chocolate

In Ayurveda, chocolate is a classic example of 'Srota Blocker'. Srotas are the 'channels' in the body that must be kept clear in order to ensure good health and vitality. When these channels are blocked, they lead to unpleasant symptoms and even major diseases. The main culprits in chocolate are the high level of carbohydrates and milk solids. You can counter the bad effect of chocolates by drinking hot water with cardamom pods. The hot water helps 'melt' the improperly digested foodstuffs and cardamom pods re-open the srotas or channels.

### Alcohol

The worst effect of excessive alcohol consumption is on the liver cells. Alcohol can produce an adverse effect on the liver functions resulting in hepatitis, alcoholic liver disease, ascites and finally liver cancer. Though the effect can not be reversed completely, a tremendous reduction in the alcoholic liver damage can be achieved through the intake of turmeric. People are advised to take 1-2 pinches of this herb in a glass of water or add it to normal cooking as a part of general routine.

Drinking hot water with a pinch of turmeric can also provide relief from hangover. The stimulating and depressing effects of alcohol can be avoided by eating 1-2 cardamom seeds or chewing a pinch of cumin seeds. Another herb that can help treat hangover is dried out Ojas. Ojas improves digestion and is believed to be the primary link between consciousness and our body. It is considered the material equivalent of bliss and gives us mental clarity and resistance to disease.

## Seafood

Seafood is 'hot' by nature and can cause problems related to digestive heat like heartburn, acid reflux, gastritis and indigestion. The best antidote to offset the effect of seafood is Peppermint Tea. It reduces the excess stomach heat and prevents the unpleasant symptoms. I think this is where the culture of eating 'peppermint' after dinner came from... though it's hard to explain where the chocolate came into the equation!!!

## Sunburn

The best antidote to relieve the symptoms of sunburn is Aloe Vera. Fresh Aloe Vera gel is highly therapeutic for a sun-damaged skin. Apply regularly to prevent skin damage and hasten repair.

## Red eyes

Soreness or redness of the eyes can occur due to a number of reasons including infections, sun exposure and overuse. An effective and time-tested antidote for the sore eyes caused due to the exposure to sun is rose water eye spray. Add 2-3 spoons of rose water in a glass of water and splash it on the eyes or eye bath with cold milk. Putting sliced cucumbers on both the eyelids can also counter the effect of harsh sun on the eyes.

## Motion sickness

Ayurveda recommends fresh ginger squeeze for reducing motion sickness. Take $1/4^{th}$ teaspoon of freshly squeezed ginger juice and add to it a little lemon juice and a pinch of salt. Simply lick the spoon dipped in this mixture to get rid of the sensation.

## Coffee

Most people will be surprised to know that excessive intake of coffee can cause unpleasant symptoms. Coffee contains caffeine, which over-stimulates the nervous system resulting in insomnia. Drinking a glass of warm milk or 2-3 glasses of warm water will counter the effect of excess caffeine in your body and will help you get a good sleep. The ill-effects of coffee can also be kept at bay by using nutmeg powder.

Besides these, there are several other substances like cheese, eggs, curd, fish and meat that can cause a negative effect on our body. Since the adverse effects of these food items are known, you can make them wholesome by combining them with the right counteracting food items or "antidotes" as given below:

- Cheese increases mucous production and congestion in the respiratory passages resulting in nose block and breathlessness. It also aggravates pitta and kapha. You can counteract this effect by adding black pepper to it.

- Eggs, in raw form, can increase kapha and in cooked form, can increase pitta. Counter this by adding turmeric or by eating raw onions with them.

- Ice-cream can cause severe breathing problems and nasal congestion. If taking ice-cream is inevitable, top it with cardamom and clove.

- Curd is also known to increase the mucous production and cause nasal congestion. Using cumin and ginger can help you take care of the ill-effects of curd.

- Legumes are known to produce gaseous distention of the abdomen. Garlic, black pepper, cloves, ginger and chili powder are the best antidotes for this.

- Fish can increase pitta. Lime, coconut and lemon are the best remedial measures to antidote the bad effects of fish.

*Chapter Eleven*

# YOGA AND AYURVEDA

Yoga is an ancient science that aims at balancing the mind for achieving self-realization and awareness. It reveals to us the secret powers of the body, mind, breath and the senses. It also unfolds the transformational methods to work on them through herbs, asana, diet, pranayama and meditation. Yoga has the power to change the lives of those who practice it regularly. Ayurveda and yoga work together for optimal health and vitality.

## Link between Yoga and ayurveda

It is quite a revelation to see how ayurveda and yoga are interrelated. Both originate from a greater system of Vedic knowledge that we can call as our nurturing mother. Ayurveda originates in the Atharva Veda and Rig Veda and Yoga originates in the Yajur Veda.

Just like ayurveda, the concepts of yoga are also based on the principles of the panchamahabuthas (earth, space, fire, air, water) and trigunas (sattva, rajas and tamas). Yoga and ayurveda encompass an understanding of how our body works and the effect of food and medicines on our body.

In treatment, ayurveda and yoga both advocate a regular practice of pranayama and meditation together with the use of herbs, following healthy diet, body purification procedures and chanting of mantras for better physical and mental health.

You can benefit from practicing a sequence of yoga posture to resolve the most excessive type of dosha (kapha, vata, pitta) in your body. This will help you to restore your body to a more balanced, serene state.

### What are the benefits of Yoga?

Peaceful mind, good health, weight loss, a strong and flexible body and a glowing beautiful skin– whatever you may be looking for, yoga can help you achieve it. Yoga is not limited to asanas (yoga poses). Its benefits can be perceived not only at the physical level; but also in uniting the mind, body and breath. When your body is in harmony with the mind and soul, the journey through life becomes much happier, calmer and more fulfilling.

- ### All-round fitness

A good health does not mean mere absence of a disease. It is a joyful, loving and enthusiastic expression of life. Yoga can help you stay physically fit and emotionally balanced. The postures, meditation and pranayama (breathing techniques) of yoga together offer a holistic fitness package.

### • Weight loss

Obesity is a very common health problem that has maximum number of medications, which promise instant miraculous results. However, people who have tried them know that weight loss can not be achieved by these so-called 'magic' pills. However, dieting - another common approach to weight loss - is not an easy approach to stick to for a long time. People tend to give in to their temptations and start binge eating just within a few days of starting their crash diet over-enthusiastically. Crash dieting and using 'magic' pills can also have several negative consequences on the health. On the other hand, Yoga offers gradual weight loss in a natural and healthy way. Kapal Bhati pranayama and Sun Salutations (Surya Namaskar) are some ways to lose weight with yoga. Regular practice of yoga can also help us become more sensitive to the type of food our body needs and when. This can help us to keep a check on the weight gain in future.

### • Stress relief

Practicing yoga for a few minutes during the day is a great way to get rid of stress. Yoga postures, meditation and pranayama are the most effective techniques for releasing mental anxieties and physical stress.

### • Inner peace

We often plan to visit serene spots, rich in natural beauty to achieve the inner peace. However, we do not realize that peace can also be found right within us. We can take our mini-vacation to experience serenity any time of the day! You can achieve the benefits of a small holiday everyday with yoga. It helps calm a disturbed mind.

### • Improved immunity

Our system is a blend of mind, spirit and body. Any unpleasantness or restlessness in the mind can manifest as a physical ailment and any irregularity in the body can affect the mind. Yoga poses strengthen the muscles, control restlessness and improve the immunity thereby preventing such irregularities.

### • Living with greater awareness

Our mind is continuously involved in one or the other activity. It keeps swinging from the past to the future; but never stays in the present. We can save ourselves from getting worked up and relax the mind by being aware of this tendency of the mind. Yoga helps us create that awareness and brings the mind back to the present, where it can stay focused.

### • Better relationships

Yoga can help you improve the relationship with your parents, spouse, friends and loved ones! A relaxed, happy and contented mind is better able to cope with sensitive relationship issues.

- **Increased energy**

We have to keep shuttling between multiple tasks throughout the day. Due to this, we feel completely drained out by the end of the day. A few minutes of yoga can uncover the secrets to feeling fresh and energetic after a long, tiring day. A 10-minute meditation while at desk can help you feel recharged in the middle of a hectic day.

- **Better posture and flexibility**

Including yoga in our daily routine can benefit the body to become flexible and supple. Regular yoga tones and stretches the body muscles and makes them strong. It also improves the body posture when you stand, sit or walk. This, in turn, can help you get rid of the ailments caused due to incorrect posture.

- **Better intuition**

Yoga has the power to improve your intuitive ability so that you can effortlessly realize what needs to be done, how and when, to yield positive results.

The Vedic system of medicine (Ayurveda) and the Vedic spiritual practice (Yoga) together form a complete approach to bring harmony and well-being to the mind, body and soul. Yoga is a continuous process. The more regular you are with your yoga practice, the more profound are its benefits. So, keep practicing!

# Chapter Twelve

# MASSAGE THERAPIES IN AYURVEDA

Ayurvedic massage creates a deep relaxation in the muscles of the body and corrects the deeply rooted imbalances in the system thereby restoring harmony and functional integrity of the doshas. Ayurvedic massage uses different types of medicated oils for inducing long, vigorous strokes throughout the body.

Ayurveda offers massage therapies that aim at keeping the enzymes in the body at their normal functioning level, thereby revitalizing the tissues and cells. A massage helps soothe the nerves and strengthens the bones. It also creates a sense of tranquility in the mind, delays the process of aging and reduces the risk of future ailments.

**Some more benefits of Ayurvedic Massage Therapies include:**

- Improves blood circulation and lymphatic drainage
- Eliminates toxins from the body
- Alleviates potential adverse effects of stress
- Stimulates the immune power and strengthens the resistance to infections
- Eases constipation, relieves abdominal spasm and aids in digestion
- Eases muscular aches and pains while promoting muscle relaxation

## Here are a few massage therapies offered in ayurveda

### • Abhyangam

Abhyangam is characterized by long strokes, Marma point therapy and flowing movements. Abhyangam is a luxurious, warm oil massage that focuses on calming the circulatory and nervous systems. This complete body massage improves the ability of nutrients to reach all the body cells and removes the stagnant waste. Concoction of warm herbal oils used in this massage nourishes and revitalizes the tissues. It heightens awareness and directs the internal healing system of the body. This treatment produces a deep healing effect by bringing harmony into the body, mind and spirit, naturally. Abhyangam is an unparalleled blissful experience.

### • Udwartanam (Herbal Anti-cellulite therapy)

Udwartanam is one of the most rejuvenating and relaxing treatments in Ayurveda. The simple procedure involves massaging the entire body below the neckline. It uses a powder prepared from an assortment of herbs in the direction opposite to the hair growth. It opens the circulatory channels and facilitates metabolic activity. It also improves the complexion of the skin and is extremely effective in reducing excess fats from the body.

- **Shirodhara**

Shirodhara awakens the mind while lulling the entire body to create a state of calmness. Stimulation and massage of the Marma points on the head, shoulders, neck and the feet is followed by warm streams of Ayurvedic oil poured on and across the forehead, continually. A deep intuitive and meditative state is awakened and a great mental clarity and shift of awareness is experienced during the treatment. Shirodhara releases stress and quiets the mind. In short, this massage therapy induces a heightened mental state and creates profound relaxation of the body.

- **Podikizhi**

Podikizhi belongs to the form of Ayurvedic therapies of high repute called Sweda. It involves the use of small linen bags that are filled with medicated powders prepared from the roots of 12 herbal plants. It is heated and applied all over the body to induce sweating. Two bundles, containing medicines and the medicated powder, are applied by 2 massage therapists to different parts of the body, simultaneously.

Podikizhi takes care of the diseases caused by disrupted Kapha and Vata doshas such as arthritis, rheumatic disorder and spondylosis. Muscular stiffness and sprain can also be prevented by undergoing this massage therapy as it tones the musculature.

- **Elakizhi**

Herbal bundles called poultices are prepared with fresh herbs and leaves as a part of this treatment. These bundles are warmed in medicated oils and used for massaging the entire body including the neck, hands, shoulders and the back while shifting the person side to side. The treatment significantly reduces chronic pain.

- **Navrakizhi**

Milk and red rice are cooked together with natural ayurvedic herbs to make a kheer or pudding. The same is later collected in Potalis or boluses and massaged over the skin. It works as an intensely invigorating therapy. It is advised for people who complain of generalized weakness and low energy. This massage is also recommended for brides-to-be as an herbal body polish.

- **Netra Basti/Netra Tarpanam**

We are constantly bombarded with strong optical stimuli due to which our eyes feel tired and strained, creating adverse effects on our vision and also on the brain's activity. Netra Basti can help prevent this by producing a soothing effect on the eyes and the surrounding tissues. The treatment includes a light facial massage that emphasizes on the Marma points around the lymph nodes and the eyes. Subsequently, dough rings are placed around each eye forming a dam. Then, the eyes are bathed in warm ayurvedic Ghee (herbal clarified butter). This nurtures and revitalizes the eyes. Later, eye exercises are performed and the Marma points on the hands are gently massaged. Thereafter, a Marma point massage for the face, neck, head and the shoulder completes the experience. This massage is ideal for people suffering from diabetes related eye problems and computer vision syndrome.

- **Griva Basti / Kati Basti**

Griva refers to the neck region, while Kati refers to the lower back and hip region. In these localized therapies, a round-shaped dam of wheat flour is sealed around the indicated area and a dough ring is filled with warm herbal oil, which is constantly replenished. Later, the dough ring is removed and the area massaged by emphasizing the Marma points. The treatment concludes with gentle stretching of the local muscles. The treatment helps to relieve pain in the local areas, especially when associated with degenerative bony changes.

- **Kavialyam**

This massage therapy is about exfoliating the skin with herbs like sesame, ginger, clove, cardamom and other powders mixed in red rice. It concludes with the application of an herbal pack that is comprised of licorice on the entire body. Licorice acts as an anti-tanning agent and helps in the removal of pigmentation.

- **Sayujyam**

This therapy involves scrubbing the body with red rice, tamarind and herbs followed by a yogurt and tamarind pack. Then, the body is covered by herbal or banana leaves to make a body wrap. Tamarind contains natural AHAs that help in the removal of tan, while yogurt helps by bleaching the skin. The synergistic effect of both makes the skin glowing and vibrant.

- **Nasyam**

In this treatment, therapists massage the upper body, from the shoulders to stimulate sweating. A dose of herbal medication is then poured into each nostril. While doing this, the area around the shoulders, nose and neck is massaged continuously. This treatment is effective in alleviating sinus, chronic colds, headaches, migraines, chest congestion and throat problems. It is also known to soothe and nourish the entire nervous system.

# Chapter Thirteen

# AYURVEDA AND MENTAL HEALTH

It's normal for any person to feel fearful or anxious, happy or sad, confused or forgetful sometimes. These are the hills and valleys of emotions that all the people experience in their daily lives. But when these emotions or thoughts frequently trouble them and cause disruption in their lives, they could be suffering from a mental illness.

According to the World Health Organization (WHO), more than 400 million people across the world are affected by psychological or behavioral problems. However, determining that a person has a mental ailment and which one it might be, is the greatest challenge psychiatrists face today because the symptoms of most of these disorders overlap.

Even though the prevalence of mental illness is as high as one in every five people, it still carries a social stigma and discrimination because of which the patients and their family members are reluctant to accept the problem and seek treatment. Unfortunately, when mental illness is left untreated, it can result in suicide. Ayurveda can provide a holistic treatment for such patients by offering them safe and natural herbal medications.

## The understanding of mental health in Ayurvedic medicine

Ayurveda views each human being as a unique combination of body, mind and spirit, including the psychology and emotions. It incorporates rejuvenation, longevity and self-realization therapies utilizing herbs, yoga, diet, breathing exercises, meditation, massage, aromas and mantras.

Ayurveda uses the concept of three doshas; vata, pitta and kapha, which when unbalanced, can affect us mentally causing disturbed emotions and thoughts. This is usually reflected at a physical level also and visa versa. Here is a list of some mental health disorders that are common today and the ayurvedic treatment for the same.

## Depression

Depression can be described as a prolonged state of sadness or a feeling of hopelessness, which is often accompanied by no highs or lows. It represents a mere bland existence that often leads to thoughts of suicide. Depression is characterized by a difficulty in doing tasks, lack of motivation, decreased appetite, short attention span, crying spells or irregular sleep pattern.

Ayurveda believes that the need to arouse the sufferer's

enthusiasm or interest in life can be achieved by introducing a sense of taste. Spices like cardamom, ginger and basil are used to open the mind and heart. Calamus teas can be given with honey and ginger. Sages and mints of all types are useful. Color therapy is often used by ayurvedic experts to elevate moods in depression patients. The therapy uses warm tones of yellow and gold to arouse a sense of positivity in the mind.

### Cutting or inflicting self-injury

Self-injury involves inflicting bodily harm on one's self that is severe enough to leave marks that last several hours or cause tissue damage. Cutting is the commonest form of self-injury. Patients may also try burning, biting, hair pulling, skin-picking, scratching and head banging as the means for inflicting self-injury. Although suicidal feelings may accompany such a behavior, it does not necessarily indicate a serious attempt to suicide. Most commonly, it is simply a mechanism for getting over an emotional distress.

Ayurveda uses nervine herbs like cayenne, Trikatu, cardamom, calamus and cloves for controlling such behaviors. The nourishing and warming effect of these herbs feed an emotional and sensitive heart. Pippali given with 1/4 teaspoon of honey every few hours is also good.

### Anxiety Disorders

These include panic attacks, post-traumatic stress disorder, obsessive-compulsive disorder, hypochondria, anger disorders and phobias. These disorders are characterized by a powerful feeling of panic together with the physical signs of fear like trembling, sweating and a racing heart for no obvious reason at all. Ayurveda considers anxiety as a Vata disorder and recommends Ashwagandha for such patients. It can be given twice a day in warm milk. Aromatherapy, using jasmine and rose, is also found to be beneficial in alleviating the anxiety.

## Eating Disorders

There are 3 types of eating disorders; bulimia nervosa, anorexia nervosa and binge eating disorder. Each of these has a different impact on the health of a person. These disorders were commonly associated with young women. However, they are now appearing in young men as well. Anorexia is characterized by a sudden, significant weight loss usually resulting from excessive dieting. Patients see themselves to be obese, irrespective of their actual weight. People with bulimia nervosa engage in cycles of binging or gorging themselves on large quantities of food and then using laxatives or purging methods like vomiting to rid the body of excess calories. It can cause strain on the bowel muscles resulting in serious complications. Repeated vomiting can cause erosion of the enamel of the teeth due to the acid coming from the stomach.

Ayurveda recommends these patients to fast on orange juice and water for the first 3-5 days initially. During this period, the bowels should be cleansed with a warm water enema once everyday. After this regimen, they can adopt an all-fruit diet for the next five days, taking 3 meals a day, comprising of juicy fruits at five hourly intervals. Thereafter, they can adopt a diet of lightly cooked vegetables, buttermilk and juicy fruits for about 10 days. Patients can also consume teas of cardamom, fresh ginger or fennel to regulate their digestion and stop vomiting.

## Attention-Deficit Hyperactivity Disorder (ADHD)

ADHD is a common behavioral disorder affecting school-age children. Children with ADHD are impulsive, hyperactive and have trouble focusing. They can not sit still, pay attention to details or concentrate.

Ayurveda advises a special diet for ADHD children to help correct the imbalance of doshas in the body. The diet should consist of fruits, vegetables and grains that are rich in natural vitamins, enzymes and minerals. Caffeine, sugar, processed food, MSG and other sugar substitutes should be eliminated from the diet. Any food containing food dyes, preservatives or other chemicals should be avoided. Herbal medications like Brahmi, Basil and Ashwagandha are recommended for improving the memory and attention span of the patients and for controlling their hyperactive and impulsive behavior.

# Chapter Fourteen

# PRANAYAM: THE SCIENCE AND ART OF BREATHING

Breath is Life!

If you have ever been to a yoga class, you must've heard endless praises of deep breathing exercises. The unique technique of diaphragmatic breathing engaging the abdominal muscles and the entire ribcage can help people prevent several disorders and be in the best health. It is the fact that the depth and the rhythm of our breath directly affect the state of our body and the mind. According to Ayurveda, breath is a carrier of Prana, the very force, which gives life to the body. In simple words - No breath, no energy and no life!

The ancient sages taught us that the "Prana", the vital source of energy circulating within us, can be channeled and cultivated through a spectrum of breathing exercises by practicing pranayam. Pranayam is a consciousness-based practice in ayurveda that regulates and controls the breath. It has a mysterious power to revitalize and soothe a tired body. It can re-energize a wavering mind or a flagging spirit. In the process, the mind is calmed and uplifted.

. . .

There are several Pranayam techniques; but we must select the appropriate one based on the individual needs. If done properly, it can offer invaluable health benefits. The seven breathing exercises in Ayurveda are explained below:

### I. **Bhastrika :**

Take deep breaths and release. Fill up your lungs fully while breathing in and force the entire breath out. Do it in a rhythm. Imagine that all the energy from the universe is entering within your body and soul. Feel that all your toxins and negativity are being expelled out. Practice this for 5 minutes once daily to stay in good health. Do this twice daily if you are ailing.

Bhastrika is beneficial in treating all kinds of skin problems including chronic disorders like leucoderma. People suffering from abnormal discoloration due to burns have also benefitted from practicing this pranayam sincerely.

### I. **Kapalbhati**

Inhale the air deeply as if taking it into your tummy and breathe out with a jerk. Make sure only your stomach moves while practicing this and not the body. Breathing out should move the Adam's apple as it pushes through the throat. You should do this for fifteen minutes daily, five minutes each, three times.

. . .

This breathing exercise helps people with cancer and other chronic conditions. These patients can practice this for 30 minutes daily. It also helps people with diabetes. It causes regeneration of the insulin producing beta cells and improves the metabolism of carbohydrates. It also improves the health of the heart by opening up the blocked arteries.

### 3. Bahya Pranayam

Take deep breaths and release. Push the stomach in completely and hold as you force the breath out. Move your head downwards till the chin touches the upper portion of the torso. Hold this position for 10-15 seconds and then move the head up and breathe in. Repeat this for about 5-11 times.

### 4. Agnisar

Take a deep breath and breathe out. Pull the stomach in while breathing out. Hold the breath for 15 seconds when you move the stomach in and out. Then breathe in again. Repeat this 3-5 times. This pranayam method helps people with digestive disorders like Irritable Bowel Syndrome, gastritis, chronic constipation and indigestion.

### 5. Anulom Bilom

Anulom Bilom is a very important pranayam method. Sit straight and close the right nostril with your thumb. Place the index finger on the forehead and breathe in deeply through the left nostril. Then, close the left nostril with the ring and little fingers joined together and breathe out through the right nostril. Then, take a deep breath through the right nostril, close it with the thumb and breathe out through the left nostril. This forms one cycle of Anulom Bilom. Repeat this cycle for five minutes. This pranayam opens all the closed channels, recharges the entire body and re-directs the flow of energy within the body.

## 6. Bhramari

Close your ears with the index finger and the middle finger. Close the eyes and rest the thumb finger on the forehead. Keep the mouth closed. Then, take a deep breath and release it through the nostrils with a loud noise from the throat. The noise should reverbate through the whole body. Repeat the exercise 5-11 times. Pranayam will relax your mind and body and activate all the glands in the head.

## 7. Udgeeth

This is a very enjoyable pranayam. Take a deep breath. Release the breath through the mouth making the sound "Om". Repeat this 5-11 times. This brings you closer to the divine element within you.

## Here are some benefits of Pranayam:

- Breath = Life. Our energy levels depend on our breath. The fuller you breathe; the more energy your body and mind will have. Taking deeper breaths also brings in more oxygen into the organs and tissues. Consider pranayam as being in an oxygen cafe!

- Deep breaths reduce stress and improve the

digestion. Slow breaths activate the parasympathetic nervous system, which gives the body a chance to regenerate, recuperate and heal.

- Pranayam helps to strengthen the immune system and improves the ability of the body to fight infections.

- Deep breaths ensure less inflammation! Most types of cancer occur as a result of inflammation. Deep breathing exercises reduce inflammation in the body thereby minimizing your risk of cancer.

- Deep breaths also improve one's awareness levels. It makes you be more aware of the present moment and helps you to connect with your intuition. Your body knows exactly what and when to feed itself to stay healthy, how much to move and how much to rest. Learning to listen to that inner voice and understanding it can help us follow what is best for the body and stay in good health.

- Slower breaths also ensure better relationships. Most relationships can be improved if people are less reactive. If you are able to step back mentally and think before talking, instead of saying something mean; you can contribute a lot to developing a positive relationship. When you are angry or frustrated, your breaths are fast and shortened. When you are calm and relaxed, the breaths are slow and complete. Pranayam teaches one to control the breath in order to control anger and allows you to look at the situation from a new perspective.

# Chapter Fifteen

# THE BENEFITS OF AYURVEDA

The healing system of ayurveda offers numerous health benefits. That is the reason people across the world are turning to this natural therapy for treating their ailments and for preventing diseases. Here are a few benefits of ayurvedic system of medicine:

- Ayurvedic medicines are prepared from pure natural herbs. They do not contain any chemicals. Hence, they are free from harmful side effects. Besides, each herb has unique medicinal properties and a pleasant flavor and aroma. These herbs act as a perfect mechanism to bring about a balanced synergy between the body, mind and spirit and promise to maintain the life indefinitely. In contrast to the synthetic drugs, these herbal medicines are considered much safer.
- Ayurvedic science does not have a disease-specific approach. Ayurveda aims at genetically determining the characteristics of the internal as well as external

features of a person instead of simply focusing on curing the disease. Herbal medicines create an internal harmony among different organs of the body and also between the body and the surrounding environment. These medicines rejuvenate the entire body system and not just treat a specific ailment.

- The holistic approach of ayurvedic herbs aids in proper absorption and digestion. They also act as an appetizer. The herbs act as a source of refreshing energy for the mind and the soul besides acting as a substitute for proteins, vitamins and essential minerals.

- The therapeutic value of ayurveda ranges in a broad spectrum and acts as a preventive medicine. It helps in the rejuvenation of the entire immune system. It enhances the energy levels in the body and enlightens the soul, mind and the cognitive organs.

- Ayurvedic medicines are highly beneficial in treating metabolic disorders without the use of hormonal supplements. The herbs act on the body as a whole and improve the co-ordination between various hormone-secreting organs to ensure correct balance of the hormones.

- The treatment works at par with the allopathic drugs in terms of relief and cure; however the relief is brought about without causing any adverse effects. Ayurveda also offers treatment for challenging diseases like cancer and AIDS.

- Herbal remedies are nutritive and self-contained rendering them non-toxic and nourishing for the body.

- Ayurveda deals with not just the medical science,

but also with the social, intellectual, ethical and spiritual aspects of the life of a person.

- Ayurvedic treatment is non-invasive in nature. It can be used as an alternative therapy or alongside other conventional therapies.
- The natural ingredients used in ayurvedic medicines are derived from herbs, plants, flowers, fruits, etc. making the therapy and the whole experience closer to the nature.
- The beneficial effect of ayurvedic treatment lasts for a longer duration in contrast to the allopathic drugs whose action lasts only for a specific duration. The result of herbal treatment is usually permanent and helps a person avoid recurrence of the illness.
- Ayurvedic medicines can be used even by healthy people as they are restorative in nature and help in enhancing mental ability and nourishment of the body.
- Ayurvedic treatment and herbal medicines are much cheaper than other systems of medicine.
- Ayurveda recommends readily available kitchen herbs and spices for minor ailments. These medicines can also be given to children and elderly patients without the fear of adverse reaction.
- Dubbed as the "science of life" or the "knowledge of life," Ayurveda can help people improve the overall quality of their life.
- A multitude of herbs in ayurveda are mixed together to combat and prevent immune disorders. These combinations are believed to help strengthen the body's defense mechanisms so that the illnesses have less chance of settling in.

The philosophy of ayurveda includes a series of conceptual systems that are characterized by health and disease, balance and disorder. Health/disease is a result of interconnectedness or the lack of it between everything that occurs in the physical, mental, emotional and spiritual being. To remain healthy, there must be a harmony between the thoughts, feelings and physical actions. Ayurvedic medications together with yoga, meditation, massage therapies and breathing exercises help people achieve this harmony and maintain optimum health. After an ayurvedic treatment, a person finds an overall improvement in their physical, mental and psychological state.